VOICE BOX SURGERY NUTRITION

A Comprehensive Guide To Optimal Surgery Recovery Nutrition, Featuring Healing Recipes, Meal Plans, And Expert Tips For Long-Term Wellness

ALLAN FREDA

1

Contents

This book focuses on the significance of nutrition in facilitating a smooth recovery process post-surgery. It delves into the intricacies of tailored dietary plans, offering healing recipes specifically designed to support the body's recovery needs. Additionally, the book provides expert insights and tips aimed at ensuring long-term wellness beyond the recovery phase. With its evidence-based approach and practical advice, this guide serves as a valuable companion for anyone navigating the challenges of voice box surgery recovery.

INTRODUCTION

Welcome to a comprehensive guide on optimal surgery recovery nutrition, specifically tailored for individuals undergoing voice box surgery.

In the realm of medical procedures, voice box surgery stands out as a significant intervention often necessitated by conditions such as cancer, trauma, or severe vocal cord dysfunction.

While the surgical process itself is crucial for addressing these health concerns, the journey to full recovery extends beyond the operating table. Nutrition plays a pivotal role in this recovery process, influencing healing, immune function, and overall well-being. In this guide, we delve into the intricacies of post-voice box surgery nutrition, offering insights, meal plans, healing recipes, and expert tips to facilitate accelerated healing and long-term wellness.

Understanding the Importance of Nutrition Post-Voice Box Surgery

Voice box surgery, also known as a laryngectomy, involves the partial or complete removal of the larynx, the organ responsible for producing sound and protecting the airway during swallowing.

This surgical procedure is often a necessary step in treating conditions such as laryngeal cancer, severe injury to the larynx, or advanced laryngeal stenosis. While the surgery is instrumental in addressing these underlying health issues, it brings about significant changes to the individual's anatomy and physiological functions, particularly in swallowing, speech production, and nutritional intake.

Nutritional Challenges Post-Voice Box Surgery

Following voice box surgery, individuals encounter various challenges related to nutrition. One of the primary concerns is dysphagia, or difficulty in swallowing, which arises due to alterations in the anatomy of the throat and the loss of protective mechanisms provided by the larynx. Dysphagia not only affects the ability to consume solid foods but also increases the risk of aspiration, where food or liquid enters the airway instead of the esophagus, leading to respiratory complications.

Additionally, the alteration in speech production post-surgery may impact the coordination of swallowing muscles, further exacerbating swallowing difficulties. These challenges necessitate modifications in dietary intake and meal consistency to ensure adequate nutrition while minimizing the risk of complications.

Key Nutrients for Healing and Recovery

Optimal nutrition post-voice box surgery is essential for supporting the healing process, bolstering immune function, and promoting overall well-being. Several key nutrients play critical roles in these aspects of recovery. Protein is paramount for tissue repair and wound healing, making it indispensable for individuals undergoing surgery. Adequate protein intake helps rebuild muscle tissue, supports immune function, and prevents muscle wasting, which may occur due to decreased physical activity during recovery.

Additionally, vitamins and minerals such as vitamin C, vitamin A, zinc, and selenium are crucial for immune support and tissue regeneration.

These micronutrients act as antioxidants, scavenging free radicals and promoting the repair of damaged cells and tissues. Furthermore, omega-3 fatty acids exhibit anti-inflammatory properties, which can aid in reducing post-operative inflammation and supporting cardiovascular health. Ensuring sufficient intake of these nutrients through a well-balanced diet is imperative for promoting optimal healing and recovery post-voice box surgery.

Strategies for Enhancing Nutritional Intake

Navigating the nutritional challenges post-voice box surgery requires strategic approaches to optimize nutrient intake while addressing swallowing difficulties and dietary restrictions.

One effective strategy is to modify the texture and consistency of foods to facilitate safe swallowing. Pureed, mashed, or soft foods are easier to swallow and less likely to cause aspiration, making them suitable options for individuals with dysphagia. Additionally, incorporating nutrient-dense liquids such as smoothies, soups, and fortified beverages can help meet calorie and nutrient needs while minimizing the risk of aspiration.

These liquids can be enriched with protein powders, fortified with vitamins and minerals, or supplemented with high-calorie ingredients to enhance their nutritional content.

Moreover, frequent, small meals and snacks spaced throughout the day can prevent fatigue and promote adequate nutrient intake without overwhelming the digestive system. Consulting with a registered dietitian or speech-language pathologist can provide personalized guidance and recommendations tailored to individual needs and preferences.

Healing Recipes and Meal Plans for Recovery

Crafting healing recipes and meal plans tailored to the specific nutritional needs and challenges post-voice box surgery can simplify the process of nourishment and support optimal recovery.

Emphasizing nutrient-dense foods that are easy to swallow, digest, and absorb is essential for meeting calorie and nutrient requirements while minimizing the risk of complications. Incorporating a variety of fruits, vegetables, whole grains, lean proteins, and healthy fats ensures a diverse array of nutrients to support healing and overall health. Sample meal plans can include options such as oatmeal with mashed bananas and almond butter for breakfast, vegetable, and lentil soup for lunch, and baked salmon with mashed sweet potatoes for dinner. Snacks can consist of yogurt with pureed fruit, smoothies made with protein powder and berries, or avocado toast on soft whole-grain bread. These recipes and meal plans provide a framework for nourishing the body post-surgery and promoting optimal healing and recovery.

In addition to dietary modifications and meal planning, incorporating expert tips and strategies can further enhance the healing process and support long-term wellness post-voice box surgery. Staying hydrated is paramount for maintaining optimal health and supporting recovery, especially in individuals with swallowing difficulties.

Sipping water frequently throughout the day, using a straw or specialized drinking cup, and avoiding dry or sticky foods can help prevent dehydration and facilitate swallowing. Engaging in gentle exercises such as swallowing exercises, neck and shoulder stretches, and diaphragmatic breathing can promote recovery, improve swallowing function, and enhance overall well-being. Moreover, seeking support from healthcare professionals, support groups, and peer mentors can provide invaluable guidance, encouragement, and emotional support throughout the recovery journey. By implementing these expert tips and strategies, individuals can accelerate healing, optimize nutrition, and achieve long-term wellness following voice box surgery.

nutrition plays a crucial role in the recovery process post-voice box surgery, influencing healing, immune function, and overall well-being. By understanding the nutritional challenges, prioritizing key nutrients, implementing strategic approaches, and incorporating healing recipes and meal plans, individuals can optimize their nutritional intake and support accelerated healing and long-term wellness. Expert tips and strategies further enhance the recovery process, promoting optimal health and quality of life following voice box surgery.

Through a holistic approach encompassing nutrition, exercise, and emotional support, individuals can navigate the journey to recovery with resilience, determination, and hope.

CHAPTER 1
PREPARING FOR SURGERY
Preparing Your Body: Nutritional Guidelines Before Surgery

Before undergoing voice box surgery, it's essential to prepare your body adequately to optimize your healing process and overall recovery. Proper nutrition plays a crucial role in this preparation phase, as it can help boost your immune system, reduce inflammation, promote tissue repair, and enhance overall well-being.

One fundamental aspect of pre-surgery nutrition is ensuring that your body is adequately nourished and hydrated. This involves consuming a balanced diet rich in essential nutrients such as vitamins, minerals, proteins, carbohydrates, and healthy fats. Adequate protein intake is particularly important, as it provides the building blocks necessary for tissue repair and wound healing.

In addition to focusing on macronutrients, it's also essential to pay attention to micronutrients, including vitamins and minerals. Vitamins C and E, for example, are known for their antioxidant properties, which can help protect cells from damage caused by free radicals and promote healing. Similarly, zinc is crucial for immune function and wound healing, making it an essential nutrient to include in your pre-surgery diet.

Hydration is another critical aspect of pre-surgery nutrition. Staying adequately hydrated can help maintain optimal blood flow, promote the elimination of toxins from the body, and support overall cellular function.

Aim to drink plenty of water throughout the day and limit your intake of dehydrating beverages such as caffeine and alcohol.

As you prepare for voice box surgery, it's essential to stock your pantry with nutritious ingredients that will support your body's healing process. Having a well-stocked pantry ensures that you have access to healthy options during your recovery period and can help you avoid the temptation of unhealthy convenience foods.

When stocking your pantry, focus on including a variety of nutrient-dense foods that will provide your body with the essential nutrients it needs to heal and recover. Some essential ingredients to consider include:

1.   Whole grains: Opt for whole grains such as brown rice, quinoa, oats, and whole wheat pasta. These foods are rich in fiber, vitamins, and minerals, providing sustained energy and promoting digestive health.

2.   Lean proteins: Choose lean sources of protein such as skinless poultry, fish, tofu,

legumes, and eggs. Protein is essential for tissue repair and muscle maintenance, making it a crucial component of your pre-surgery diet.

3.	Fruits and veggies: Include a range of vibrant fruits and vegetables in your diet. to ensure you're getting a wide range of vitamins, minerals, and antioxidants.

4.	Aim to fill half of your plate with fruits and vegetables at each meal to maximize your nutrient intake.

5.	Healthy fats: Include sources of healthy fats such as avocados, nuts, seeds, and olive oil in your pantry. These fats are essential for cell membrane function, hormone production, and nutrient absorption, and can help reduce inflammation in the body.

6.	Herbs and spices: Stock up on herbs and spices to add flavor to your meals without relying on excess salt or unhealthy condiments. Herbs and spices such as garlic, ginger, turmeric, and cinnamon also have anti-inflammatory properties, which can support your body's healing process.

By stocking your pantry with these essential ingredients, you'll be well-prepared to nourish your body before voice box surgery and support optimal healing and recovery. Additionally, having a variety of nutritious options on hand will make it easier to adhere to your pre-surgery dietary guidelines and maintain overall health and well-being.

☐

CHAPTER 2
RECOVERY NUTRITION
BASICS

In the realm of post-surgery care, nutrition plays a pivotal role in facilitating the healing process and ensuring optimal recovery. As the body undergoes the rigors of surgery, it demands a specialized blend of nutrients to repair tissues, boost the immune system, and regain strength. Understanding the fundamentals of recovery nutrition is paramount in promoting faster healing, reducing the risk of complications, and enhancing long-term wellness.

Fueling Your Recovery: Essential Nutrients and Their Roles

In the aftermath of voice box surgery, the body's nutritional needs undergo a significant shift. Essential nutrients such as protein, carbohydrates, fats, vitamins, and minerals play indispensable roles in supporting the healing process. Protein, often hailed as the building blocks of tissue, is particularly crucial for repairing damaged cells and promoting muscle recovery. Adequate intake of carbohydrates replenishes glycogen stores, providing the body with the energy it needs to fuel various physiological processes and combat post-surgical fatigue. Healthy fats, including omega-3 fatty acids, aid in reducing inflammation and supporting immune function.

Moreover, a spectrum of vitamins and minerals, ranging from vitamin C and zinc to calcium and magnesium, are instrumental in bolstering the immune system, fortifying bones, and facilitating cellular repair. Balancing these nutrients through a well-rounded diet is essential for optimizing recovery and minimizing the risk of nutrient deficiencies.

The Healing Power of Whole Foods: Incorporating Nutrient-Dense Ingredients

Embracing a diet rich in whole, nutrient-dense foods is a cornerstone of effective post-surgery nutrition.

Whole foods, such as fruits, vegetables, lean proteins, whole grains, and healthy fats, boast an array of vitamins, minerals, antioxidants, and phytonutrients that promote healing and enhance overall well-being. Incorporating a vibrant assortment of colorful fruits and vegetables not only provides essential vitamins and minerals but also delivers potent antioxidants that combat oxidative stress and inflammation.

Lean sources of protein, such as poultry, fish, tofu, beans, and lentils, supply the amino acids necessary for tissue repair and muscle regeneration. Whole grains, such as quinoa, brown rice, and oats, offer complex carbohydrates for sustained energy release and fiber for digestive health.

Additionally, healthy fats sourced from avocados, nuts, seeds, and olive oil contribute to cardiovascular health and possess anti-inflammatory properties. By prioritizing whole foods in post-surgery meal planning, individuals can harness the healing power of nature's bounty to expedite recovery and fortify their bodies against future health challenges.

Hydration Matters: The Importance of Fluids in Recovery

Amidst the focus on solid foods, the significance of hydration in the recovery process should not be overlooked. Proper hydration is essential for maintaining cellular function, regulating body temperature, flushing out toxins, and facilitating nutrient transport throughout the body. Dehydration can impede the healing process, exacerbate post-surgical complications, and prolong recovery time.

In the wake of voice box surgery, individuals may encounter challenges in swallowing or experience discomfort when consuming liquids. In such cases, opting for hydrating foods with high water content, such as soups, broths, smoothies, and fruits like watermelon and cucumbers, can help meet fluid needs while minimizing discomfort.

Additionally, sipping on water throughout the day and avoiding caffeinated or sugary beverages can support optimal hydration levels. Monitoring urine color and output can serve as a simple yet effective gauge of hydration status, with pale yellow urine indicating adequate hydration. By prioritizing hydration alongside nutrient-dense foods, individuals can create an optimal environment for healing, ensuring a smoother recovery journey and long-term wellness.

CHAPTER 3
SOFT AND SOOTHING RECIPES

When undergoing voice box surgery, nutrition plays a crucial role in the recovery process. A comprehensive guide to optimal surgery recovery nutrition encompasses a variety of aspects, including soft and soothing recipes designed to aid in the healing journey. These recipes are tailored to provide nourishment while being gentle on the throat and facilitating easy swallowing, promoting accelerated healing and long-term wellness.

Soft and Soothing Recipes

Soft and soothing recipes are essential for individuals recovering from voice box surgery as they offer gentle nourishment without causing discomfort or irritation to the throat. These recipes are carefully crafted to provide essential nutrients while being easy to consume, ensuring that the body receives the fuel it needs to heal efficiently.

By focusing on soft and soothing textures, these recipes help alleviate the discomfort often associated with post-surgery recovery, allowing individuals to maintain proper nutrition without exacerbating any pain or inflammation.

Gentle and Nourishing Soups for Sore Throats

Soups are a staple in post-surgery recovery nutrition due to their comforting warmth and easy-to-swallow consistency. When preparing soups for individuals recovering from voice box surgery, it's important to focus on gentle and nourishing ingredients that provide essential nutrients without irritating the throat. Opting for smooth, pureed soups or broth-based varieties can help ensure easy swallowing while still delivering vital vitamins, minerals, and hydration. Incorporating ingredients such as soft vegetables, lean proteins, and whole grains can further enhance the nutritional value of soups, promoting healing and overall wellness.

Creamy Blends: Smoothies and Shakes for Easy Swallowing

Smoothies and shakes are excellent options for individuals recovering from voice box surgery, as they offer a convenient way to consume nutrient-dense ingredients in an easily digestible form. When creating creamy blends for post-surgery nutrition, it's important to prioritize ingredients that are soft, smooth, and easy to swallow. Incorporating fruits such as bananas, berries, and mangoes can add natural sweetness and provide essential vitamins and antioxidants. Additionally, adding protein sources such as Greek yogurt, silken tofu, or protein powder can help support muscle repair and recovery. To further enhance the nutritional value of smoothies and shakes, consider adding healthy fats from sources like avocado or nut butter, as well as supplements such as collagen or probiotics to support overall healing and immune function.

Comforting Porridges and Congees: Sustaining Your Strength

Porridges and congees are traditional comfort foods that offer warmth and sustenance, making them ideal choices for individuals recovering from voice box surgery. These soft and easily digestible dishes provide a comforting way to nourish the body while promoting healing and strength. When preparing porridges and congees for post-surgery nutrition, consider using gentle grains such as rice, oats, or quinoa, which can be cooked to a smooth and creamy consistency. Adding in flavorful ingredients such as ginger, garlic, and herbs not only enhances the taste but also provides additional nutritional benefits and aids in digestion. Including soft vegetables, lean proteins, and healthy fats can further enhance the nutrient profile of these dishes, ensuring that individuals receive the essential nutrients needed for optimal recovery and long-term wellness.

soft and soothing recipes play a crucial role in post-voice box surgery nutrition, providing gentle nourishment to support healing and recovery. By incorporating ingredients that are easy to swallow and gentle on the throat, such as those found in soups, smoothies, shakes, porridges, and congees, individuals can ensure that their nutritional needs are met without causing discomfort or irritation. Additionally, focusing on nutrient-dense ingredients and incorporating a variety of flavors and textures can help promote accelerated healing and long-term wellness.

CHAPTER 4
PROTEIN-RICH DISHES

When undergoing voice box surgery, proper nutrition plays a critical role in the recovery process. Among the key nutrients, protein stands out as essential for tissue repair, wound healing, and overall immune function. In this comprehensive guide to optimal surgery recovery nutrition, we delve into the significance of protein-rich dishes, offering a variety of options tailored to different dietary preferences and needs. Whether you're a meat-eater, vegetarian, or vegan, there are ample opportunities to boost your protein intake and support your body's healing journey.

Tender Proteins: Easy to Swallow Meat and Fish Recipes

For individuals recovering from voice box surgery, consuming tender proteins is crucial, as swallowing may initially be challenging. Incorporating easy-to-swallow meat and fish recipes into your diet not only ensures an adequate protein intake but also promotes comfort during meals.

Opt for lean cuts of meat such as chicken breast, turkey, or tender cuts of beef, which can be cooked to a soft, moist consistency to facilitate swallowing. Similarly, fish varieties like salmon, tilapia, or flounder offer a rich source of protein and healthy omega-3 fatty acids, aiding in inflammation reduction and tissue repair. When preparing these dishes, consider methods such as baking, poaching, or slow-cooking to achieve optimal tenderness without compromising nutritional quality. Experiment with flavorful herbs, spices, and marinades to enhance taste while maintaining ease of swallowing.

Plant-Based Protein Power: Nourishing Dishes for Vegetarians and Vegans

For those following a vegetarian or vegan diet, plant-based protein sources provide ample nutrition to support post-surgery recovery. Incorporating nourishing dishes rich in legumes, nuts, seeds, and soy products ensures an adequate intake of essential amino acids vital for tissue regeneration and immune function. Lentils, chickpeas, black beans, and tofu are excellent sources of plant-based protein, versatile enough to be incorporated into various recipes such as soups, salads, stir-fries, and casseroles.

Additionally, quinoa, a complete protein grain, serves as a wholesome base for nutrient-packed bowls or side dishes. When preparing plant-based meals, focus on incorporating a diverse range of ingredients to maximize nutritional diversity and enhance overall healing potential.

Experiment with different cooking techniques and flavor profiles to create satisfying dishes that cater to your dietary preferences and promote optimal recovery.

Boosting Protein Intake: Tips and Tricks for Incorporating Protein Supplements

In some cases, individuals recovering from voice box surgery may struggle to meet their protein requirements through diet alone. In such instances, incorporating protein supplements can be a convenient and effective way to boost protein intake and support the healing process. Whey protein, derived from milk, is a popular choice due to its high biological value and rapid absorption rate, making it ideal for promoting muscle repair and growth. For those with lactose intolerance or dairy allergies, plant-based protein powders made from sources such as peas, rice, or hemp offer viable alternatives. These supplements can be easily added to smoothies, shakes, or homemade protein bars for a quick and convenient protein boost. When choosing protein supplements, opt for products free from added sugars, artificial flavors, and unnecessary additives to ensure optimal nutritional quality. Additionally, consult with a healthcare professional or registered dietitian to determine the appropriate dosage and timing of protein supplementation based on individual needs and recovery goals.

prioritizing protein-rich dishes is essential for promoting optimal recovery and long-term wellness following voice box surgery.

Whether opting for tender meat and fish recipes, nourishing plant-based dishes, or incorporating protein supplements, focusing on adequate protein intake supports tissue repair, wound healing, and overall immune function. By incorporating a variety of protein sources into your diet and experimenting with different recipes and cooking techniques, you can enhance the healing process and lay the foundation for sustained health and well-being.

CHAPTER 5
CARB CONSCIOUS CREATIONS

Carbohydrates serve as a primary source of energy for the body, making them an essential component of post-voice box surgery nutrition.

However, it's crucial to be mindful of the types and quantities of carbs consumed during recovery to support healing while managing potential side effects such as difficulty swallowing or chewing. This section, "Carb Conscious Creations," focuses on providing nutritious and easily digestible carbohydrate options to aid in the recovery process.

Energizing Grains: Soft and Satisfying Grain-Based Recipes

Incorporating grains into the post-voice box surgery diet can provide essential nutrients such as fiber, vitamins, and minerals while offering a comforting and satisfying texture.

Opting for soft and easily digestible grains is essential to prevent discomfort and aid in the healing process. Quinoa, amaranth, and millet are excellent choices due to their soft texture and high nutritional value. Recipes such as creamy quinoa porridge or millet pilaf can be prepared with added broth or coconut milk for extra moisture and flavor.

These grain-based dishes not only provide energy but also contribute to overall nutrition, supporting the body's recovery efforts.

Starchy Staples: Mashed and Pureed Potatoes, Sweet Potatoes, and More

Potatoes and sweet potatoes are versatile starchy staples that can be easily modified to suit the needs of individuals recovering from voice box surgery. Mashing or pureeing these root vegetables creates a soft and creamy texture that is gentle on the throat and easy to swallow.

Adding herbs, spices, or a touch of olive oil enhances the flavor while providing additional nutrients. Sweet potato mash with cinnamon and nutmeg or creamy mashed potatoes with chives are examples of comforting and nourishing dishes that can be included in the post-surgery meal plan. These starchy staples not only provide carbohydrates for energy but also offer essential vitamins and minerals crucial for healing and recovery.

Creative Carb Ideas: Reinventing Bread, Pasta, and Rice for Easy Eating

Traditional bread, pasta, and rice may pose challenges for individuals recovering from voice box surgery due to their texture and difficulty in swallowing. However, with a bit of creativity, these carb-rich staples can be reinvented into softer and more easily digestible alternatives. Opting for whole grain or gluten-free bread that is thinly sliced and lightly toasted can make it easier to chew and swallow. Similarly, using spiralized vegetables such as zucchini or sweet potato instead of traditional pasta provides a softer texture while adding extra nutrients. Additionally, replacing white rice with quinoa or cauliflower rice offers a softer consistency while boosting the dish's nutritional value. Experimenting with creative carb ideas allows individuals to enjoy their favorite foods while supporting their recovery journey.

By focusing on carb-conscious creations such as energizing grains, starchy staples, and creative carb ideas, individuals can ensure they meet their nutritional needs while promoting healing and recovery after voice box surgery. These recipes and meal ideas offer a balance of carbohydrates, vitamins, and minerals essential for optimal recovery and long-term wellness. Additionally, incorporating soft and easily digestible carb options helps minimize discomfort and supports overall well-being during the recovery process.

CHAPTER 6

VITAMIN-PACKED SIDES AND SNACKS

When it comes to recovering from voice box surgery, nutrition plays a crucial role in facilitating healing, reducing inflammation, and supporting overall well-being. One essential aspect of post-operative nutrition is ensuring an adequate intake of vitamins and minerals, which are vital for tissue repair and immune function. Incorporating vitamin-packed sides and snacks into your diet can help optimize your recovery process, providing essential nutrients to support healing and enhance your overall health.

Colorful Vegetable Medleys: Roasted, Steamed, and Pureed Veggies

Vegetables are rich in vitamins, minerals, antioxidants, and fiber, making them an excellent choice for promoting healing and supporting overall health during recovery from voice box surgery.

Colorful vegetable medleys offer a diverse array of nutrients, with each hue representing different phytonutrients that contribute to various aspects of health. Roasting, steaming, or pureeing vegetables can help enhance their flavor and texture, making them easier to consume, especially if you experience any difficulty with swallowing or chewing post-surgery.

Roasting vegetables intensifies their natural flavors and caramelizes their sugars, resulting in a deliciously savory and slightly sweet taste.

Popular vegetables for roasting include carrots, sweet potatoes, bell peppers, zucchini, and cauliflower. Simply toss them with a drizzle of olive oil, sprinkle with herbs and spices, and roast in the oven until tender and golden brown.

Steaming vegetables preserve their natural color, flavor, and nutritional content while maintaining their crisp texture. Steamed vegetables are gentle on the digestive system and easy to digest, making them ideal for individuals recovering from surgery. Common vegetables for steaming include broccoli, green beans, asparagus, and Brussels sprouts. Simply steam them until fork-tender, then season with a dash of sea salt and a squeeze of lemon juice for added flavor.

Pureed vegetables provide a smooth and creamy texture that is easy to swallow and digest, making them suitable for individuals with swallowing difficulties or those transitioning to solid foods after surgery. You can puree a variety of vegetables, such as carrots, squash, spinach, and peas, either individually or in combination, to create flavorful and nutrient-rich purees. Add vegetable broth, herbs, and spices to enhance the taste and nutritional value of pureed vegetables.

Incorporating colorful vegetable medleys into your post-surgery diet can help boost your intake of essential vitamins and minerals, including vitamin A, vitamin C, vitamin K, folate, and potassium, which are crucial for supporting immune function, promoting tissue repair, and reducing inflammation. Experiment with different cooking methods and flavor combinations to create delicious and nourishing vegetable dishes that will support your recovery and enhance your overall well-being.

Fruitful Bites: Soft and Sweet Snacks for a Nutrient Boost

Fruits are nature's candy, packed with vitamins, minerals, antioxidants, and fiber, making them an excellent choice for satisfying your sweet tooth while providing essential nutrients to support your recovery from voice box surgery. Soft and sweet fruits are particularly suitable for individuals with swallowing difficulties or those who need to consume foods that are easy to chew and digest post-surgery.

Soft fruits such as bananas, avocados, ripe mangoes, and papayas are naturally creamy and easy to eat, making them ideal for snacking or incorporating into smoothies and purees.

These fruits are rich in vitamins, minerals, and healthy fats, including potassium, vitamin C, vitamin E, and folate, which are essential for supporting immune function, promoting tissue repair, and reducing inflammation.

Sweet fruits such as berries, melons, grapes, and kiwis are bursting with flavor and nutritional goodness, making them a delicious and refreshing snack option during your recovery period.

These fruits are rich in vitamins, minerals, antioxidants, and phytonutrients, which help protect cells from damage, support immune function, and promote overall health and well-being.

Incorporating fruitful bites into your post-surgery diet can help increase your intake of essential vitamins and minerals, including vitamin C, vitamin E, potassium, and antioxidants, which are crucial for supporting immune function, enhancing wound healing, and reducing the risk of infection. Enjoy fresh fruits on their own as a snack, or pair them with protein-rich foods such as Greek yogurt or nut butter for a balanced and satisfying treat.

Homemade Nut and Seed Blends: Healthy Fats for Healing

Nuts and seeds are nutrient-dense foods rich in healthy fats, protein, fiber, vitamins, minerals, and antioxidants, making them an excellent choice for promoting healing and supporting overall health during recovery from voice box surgery. Homemade nut and seed blends offer a convenient and versatile way to incorporate these nutritious ingredients into your post-operative diet, providing essential nutrients to support tissue repair, reduce inflammation, and boost immune function.

Creating your own nut and seed blends allows you to customize the flavor and nutritional profile to suit your preferences and dietary needs. You can combine a variety of nuts and seeds such as almonds, walnuts, cashews, pistachios, pumpkin seeds, sunflower seeds, and chia seeds to create a delicious and nutrient-rich blend that can be enjoyed on its own as a snack or used as a topping for yogurt, oatmeal, salads, or smoothie bowls.

Nuts and seeds are rich in heart-healthy monounsaturated and polyunsaturated fats, which help reduce inflammation, lower cholesterol levels, and support cardiovascular health. They are also excellent sources of plant-based protein, which is essential for supporting muscle repair and recovery after surgery. Additionally, nuts and seeds provide a wide range of vitamins and minerals, including vitamin E, magnesium, zinc, and selenium, which play key roles in immune function, antioxidant defense, and wound healing.

Incorporating homemade nut and seed blends into your post-surgery diet can help increase your intake of essential nutrients, including healthy fats, protein, fiber, vitamins, and minerals, which are crucial for supporting optimal healing and long-term wellness.

Enjoy a handful of nut and seed blend as a satisfying snack, or use it to add crunch and flavor to your favorite dishes for a nourishing and delicious boost. Experiment with different nut and seed combinations and flavorings to create unique blends that will support your recovery and enhance your overall health and well-being.

CHAPTER 7
FLAVORFUL SEASONINGS AND SAUCES

When it comes to post-surgery nutrition, flavor plays a crucial role in ensuring that patients enjoy their meals while also supporting their recovery process. Seasonings and sauces are essential components in adding taste and variety to dishes, particularly for those with altered palates or restricted diets following surgery. In this section, we delve into the significance of flavorful seasonings and sauces, exploring safe options for post-surgery consumption, their role in enhancing meal palatability, and strategies for incorporating a balance of sweet, sour, and savory flavors into recovery diets.

The Spice of Life: Safe and Savory Seasonings for Post-Surgery Palates

Following surgery, patients may experience changes in taste preferences or heightened sensitivity to certain flavors. However, incorporating seasonings into meals can help alleviate blandness and enhance the overall dining experience. It is essential to prioritize safe and gentle seasonings that do not irritate the digestive system or interfere with healing processes.

Herbs such as parsley, cilantro, and basil offer freshness and aroma without overwhelming the palate, making them ideal choices for seasoning post-surgery meals. Additionally, spices like ginger and turmeric possess anti-inflammatory properties, which can aid in reducing post-operative inflammation and promoting healing.

When selecting seasonings, it's crucial to avoid those high in sodium or MSG, as excessive salt intake may lead to fluid retention and hinder recovery. Opting for natural herbs and spices not only adds flavor but also contributes to the overall nutritional value of meals, supporting the body's healing process.

Savory Sauces and Dips: Adding Flavor and Moisture to Meals

Sauces and dips are versatile components that can transform simple dishes into flavorful culinary creations. For individuals recovering from surgery, sauces play a vital role in adding moisture and enhancing the palatability of meals, particularly for those with dry mouth or difficulty swallowing. When choosing sauces for post-surgery nutrition, it's essential to opt for options that are not only flavorful but also nutrient-dense and easy to digest. Homemade sauces using fresh ingredients allow for greater control over the flavor profile and nutritional content, minimizing the use of additives or preservatives that may be detrimental to recovery. Tomato-based sauces infused with herbs such as oregano and thyme offer a burst of flavor while providing essential vitamins and antioxidants. Similarly, creamy sauces made from Greek yogurt or avocado provide a smooth texture and richness without the need for excessive amounts of fat or salt. Incorporating savory sauces and dips into post-surgery meals not only enhances taste but also promotes adequate hydration and nutrient absorption, supporting the body's healing process.

Achieving a balance of sweet and sour flavors is essential in creating well-rounded post-surgery meals that satisfy the palate without overwhelming sensitive taste buds. Incorporating acidic and tangy elements into dishes can help cut through richness and add depth of flavor, enhancing the overall dining experience. However, it's crucial to select options that are gentle on the digestive system and do not exacerbate post-operative symptoms such as acid reflux or indigestion. Citrus fruits such as lemon and lime add brightness and acidity to dishes without the need for excessive amounts of salt or sugar, making them ideal for enhancing flavor while promoting hydration and vitamin C intake. Additionally, incorporating naturally sweet ingredients such as honey or maple syrup can help balance out tangy flavors and add complexity to savory dishes. When incorporating sweet and sour elements into post-surgery nutrition, moderation is key to avoiding potential gastrointestinal discomfort or blood sugar fluctuations. By carefully balancing acidic and tangy flavors, patients can enjoy a diverse range of flavorful meals that support their recovery journey while promoting long-term health and wellness.

CHAPTER 8
EASY-TO-SWALLOW
DESSERTS

After undergoing voice box surgery, it is crucial to prioritize nutrition to support the body's healing process and overall well-being. One aspect of post-surgery nutrition that often requires attention is the texture of the foods consumed.

Easy-to-swallow desserts play a significant role in providing comfort and nourishment during recovery. These desserts are designed to be gentle on the throat and easy to consume, while still offering delicious flavors and essential nutrients.

In this guide, we'll explore various options for easy-to-swallow desserts, including soft and silky puddings, decadent smooth custards, and gelatin delights, along with tips for incorporating them into a balanced post-surgery diet.

Soft and silky puddings are perfect for those recovering from voice box surgery, as they provide a smooth and creamy texture that is easy to swallow. These indulgent treats offer a comforting experience while also delivering essential nutrients to support healing. Puddings can be made with a variety of ingredients, including milk, eggs, and flavorings such as vanilla or chocolate.

They can also be enriched with additional protein and vitamins to promote recovery. When preparing puddings for post-surgery consumption, it's essential to ensure they are smooth and free from any lumps or chunks that could pose a choking hazard. By incorporating soft and silky puddings into the recovery diet, patients can enjoy a satisfying dessert while supporting their nutritional needs.

Decadent smooth custards offer a luxurious dessert option for individuals recovering from voice box surgery. With their velvety texture and rich flavor, custards provide a satisfying way to indulge in something sweet while prioritizing ease of swallowing. Like puddings, custards can be made with ingredients such as eggs, milk, and sugar, with additional flavorings such as vanilla or fruit puree. By incorporating smooth custards into the post-surgery diet, patients can enjoy a delightful dessert experience without compromising on nutrition or comfort. It's important to ensure that custards are free from any lumps or chunks and are served at an appropriate temperature to prevent discomfort during consumption. With their versatility and appeal, smooth custards make an excellent addition to a well-rounded recovery nutrition plan.

Gelatin Delights: Refreshing and Light Desserts for a Sweet Finish

Gelatin Delights offers a refreshing and light dessert option for individuals recovering from voice box surgery. These desserts are made with gelatin, which provides a jiggly texture that is easy to swallow and gentle on the throat. Gelatin can be flavored with a variety of ingredients, including fruit juices, purees, or extracts, to create delicious and nutritious treats. Additionally, gelatin is a good source of protein, which is essential for supporting the body's healing process post-surgery.

By incorporating gelatin delights into the recovery diet, patients can enjoy a sweet finish to their meals while also receiving the nutritional benefits of this versatile ingredient. It's important to ensure that gelatin desserts are properly set and chilled before serving to achieve the desired texture and consistency. With their lightness and versatility, gelatin delights offer a delightful way to satisfy sweet cravings during the recovery period.

easy-to-swallow desserts such as soft and silky puddings, decadent smooth custards, and gelatin delights play a crucial role in supporting recovery and providing comfort for individuals undergoing voice box surgery. By incorporating these delicious and nutritious options into the post-surgery diet, patients can enjoy satisfying desserts while promoting healing and long-term wellness. With careful attention to texture and ingredients, easy-to-swallow desserts can contribute to a balanced and enjoyable recovery nutrition plan.

CHAPTER 9
TROUBLESHOOTING AND TIPS

In the journey towards recovery from voice box surgery, nutrition plays a pivotal role in fostering optimal healing and long-term wellness. However, the process of maintaining a balanced diet post-surgery may present various challenges.

To aid in this endeavor, it's essential to implement strategies to overcome eating challenges, streamline meal planning, and navigate any dietary restrictions effectively. By addressing these aspects comprehensively, individuals undergoing voice box surgery can optimize their recovery journey and enhance their overall well-being.

Overcoming Eating Challenges: Strategies for Success:

Voice box surgery can significantly impact an individual's ability to swallow, chew, or digest food comfortably. Consequently, eating challenges such as dysphagia (difficulty swallowing), dysphonia (voice disorders), or dysphonia (hoarseness) may arise, hindering the intake of essential nutrients. To overcome these challenges, several strategies can be employed:

Firstly, adapting the texture of food is paramount. Opting for softer, pureed, or mashed varieties can facilitate easier swallowing and digestion, reducing the risk of discomfort or aspiration. Incorporating nutritious soups, smoothies, or protein shakes can serve as viable options to ensure adequate nutrient intake while catering to altered swallowing abilities.

Moreover, pacing during meals is crucial. Taking smaller, more frequent meals throughout the day, rather than consuming large portions in one sitting, can alleviate strain on the throat muscles and aid in efficient digestion.

Additionally, chewing food thoroughly and consciously can enhance the process of breaking down food particles, promoting smoother swallowing and reducing the likelihood of choking or discomfort.

In instances where swallowing difficulties persist, consulting with a speech therapist or dietitian specialized in dysphagia management is advisable. These professionals can offer personalized exercises, techniques, or dietary modifications tailored to individual needs, facilitating the gradual improvement of swallowing function and overall nutritional status.

Furthermore, incorporating foods rich in moisture, such as fruits, vegetables, and broths, can help alleviate dryness and irritation in the throat, promoting greater comfort during eating. Hydration is also paramount, as adequate water intake can prevent dehydration and support optimal recovery post-surgery.

Overall, adopting a patient-centered approach and being mindful of individual needs and preferences is key to overcoming eating challenges effectively post-voice box surgery. By implementing these strategies and seeking professional guidance when needed, individuals can navigate the recovery process with greater ease and promote overall well-being.

Meal Planning Made Easy: Tips for Preparation and Portioning:

Meal planning post-voice box surgery is essential to ensure a consistent intake of nutrients while minimizing discomfort and maximizing convenience. By employing practical tips for preparation and portioning, individuals can streamline the meal planning process and facilitate adherence to dietary recommendations:

Begin by establishing a diverse repertoire of nutritious recipes that align with post-surgery dietary guidelines. Focus on incorporating a balance of lean proteins, whole grains, fruits, vegetables, and healthy fats to meet nutritional needs adequately. Experimenting with different flavors, textures, and cooking methods can add variety and enjoyment to meals while catering to individual preferences.

When preparing meals, prioritize simplicity and ease of consumption. Opt for recipes that require minimal chewing or manipulation, such as casseroles, stir-fries, or one-pot dishes. Utilizing kitchen appliances such as blenders, food processors, or slow cookers can further simplify meal preparation and ensure consistency in texture and flavor.

Consider batch cooking and portioning meals in advance to streamline the eating process and minimize daily cooking efforts. Divide prepared meals into individual servings and store them in portion-sized containers for convenient access throughout the week.

Labeling containers with the date and contents can aid in organization and prevent food waste.

Additionally, incorporate nutrient-dense snacks into meal planning to sustain energy levels and prevent excessive hunger between meals. Portable options such as nuts, seeds, yogurt, or cut fruits and vegetables can serve as convenient and nutritious choices for on-the-go consumption.

Furthermore, involve family members or caregivers in the meal planning and preparation process to distribute responsibilities and foster a supportive environment. Communicate any dietary restrictions or preferences clearly to ensure that meals are tailored to individual needs and preferences effectively.

By implementing these practical tips for meal planning, individuals undergoing voice box surgery can streamline the eating process, optimize nutrient intake, and promote overall well-being during the recovery period and beyond.

Navigating Dietary Restrictions: Catering to Individual Needs:

Voice box surgery may necessitate temporary or permanent dietary restrictions to accommodate changes in swallowing function, vocal capabilities, or nutritional requirements.

Navigating these restrictions effectively involves understanding individual needs, preferences, and limitations while prioritizing nutritional adequacy and overall well-being.

Firstly, it's essential to consult with healthcare professionals, including speech therapists, dietitians, or surgeons, to ascertain specific dietary recommendations based on the nature and extent of the surgery. These professionals can provide invaluable guidance regarding texture modifications, swallowing exercises, and dietary adjustments tailored to individual circumstances.

Adhering to prescribed dietary modifications, such as soft or pureed foods, thickened liquids, or avoidance of certain food textures, is paramount to prevent complications such as aspiration or choking and promote safe swallowing post-surgery. Experimenting with alternative ingredients, cooking techniques, or flavor enhancements can help maintain variety and enjoyment in meals while adhering to dietary restrictions.

Moreover, being proactive in identifying potential allergens, intolerances, or sensitivities is crucial to prevent adverse reactions and promote gastrointestinal comfort. Reading food labels diligently, communicating dietary restrictions to food service providers, and opting for whole, minimally processed foods can aid in avoiding common allergens and irritants effectively.

In cases where dietary restrictions pose challenges in meeting nutritional needs adequately, incorporating oral nutritional supplements or fortified foods may be warranted to bridge nutrient gaps and support overall health and recovery. Collaborating with healthcare professionals to monitor nutritional status regularly and adjust dietary recommendations accordingly is essential to ensure optimal outcomes.

Additionally, fostering open communication with family members, caregivers, or dining companions regarding dietary restrictions and preferences can facilitate a supportive and inclusive dining environment. Educating others about the importance of adhering to dietary guidelines and accommodating individual needs can promote understanding and cooperation in meal preparation and consumption.

By navigating dietary restrictions effectively and prioritizing nutritional adequacy and overall well-being, individuals undergoing voice box surgery can optimize their recovery journey and enhance their quality of life in the long term.

overcoming eating challenges, streamlining meal planning, and navigating dietary restrictions are integral aspects of promoting optimal recovery and long-term wellness post-voice box surgery.

By implementing practical strategies, seeking professional guidance, and fostering a supportive environment, individuals can enhance their nutritional intake, minimize discomfort, and promote overall well-being during the recovery process and beyond.

CONCLUSION

the journey towards optimal surgery recovery nutrition is an intricate yet vital aspect of postoperative care, particularly in cases such as voice box surgery where maintaining proper nutrition is crucial. Through this comprehensive guide, we've explored the importance of nutrition in the recovery process and provided valuable insights, recipes, and meal plans to facilitate accelerated healing and long-term wellness.

Starting with the preparation phase, we emphasized the significance of pre-surgery nutritional guidelines and stocking essential pantry items to ensure a strong foundation for the recovery journey. Throughout the recovery process, we delved into the basics of recovery nutrition, emphasizing the roles of essential nutrients and the healing power of whole foods, alongside the importance of hydration.

Our exploration of soft and soothing recipes, protein-rich dishes, carb-conscious creations, vitamin-packed sides and snacks, flavorful seasonings and sauces, and easy-to-swallow desserts offered a diverse array of options catered to varying dietary needs and preferences. From gentle soups to indulgent treats, each recipe and meal idea was crafted to nourish the body and soothe the palate during the recovery period.

Moreover, our troubleshooting and tips section provided invaluable guidance on overcoming eating challenges, simplifying meal planning, and navigating dietary restrictions, ensuring that individuals can tailor their recovery nutrition journey to meet their specific needs and circumstances.

As we bid farewell to this guide, let us carry forward the knowledge and insights gained, recognizing that optimal nutrition is not merely a component of recovery but a cornerstone of overall health and well-being. May this guide serve as a beacon of support and empowerment for all those embarking on their journey to recovery, fostering resilience, healing, and vitality every step of the way.